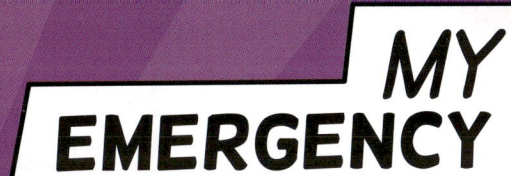

AUTISTIC MELTDOWN

By Charis Mather

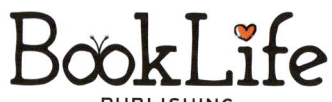

©This edition published in 2024.
First published in 2022.
**BookLife Publishing Ltd.
King's Lynn, Norfolk
PE30 4LS, UK**

All rights reserved.
Printed in India.

A catalogue record for this book is available from the British Library.

PB ISBN: 978-1-80505-675-1
HB ISBN: 978-1-80155-628-6

Written by:
Charis Mather

Edited by:
Robin Twiddy

Designed by:
Drue Rintoul

All facts, statistics, web addresses and URLs in this book were verified as valid and accurate at time of writing. No responsibility for any changes to external websites or references can be accepted by either the author or publisher. The contents of this book are intended as solely informative and should not be considered medical advice. BookLife recommends contacting medical professionals for specific guidance.

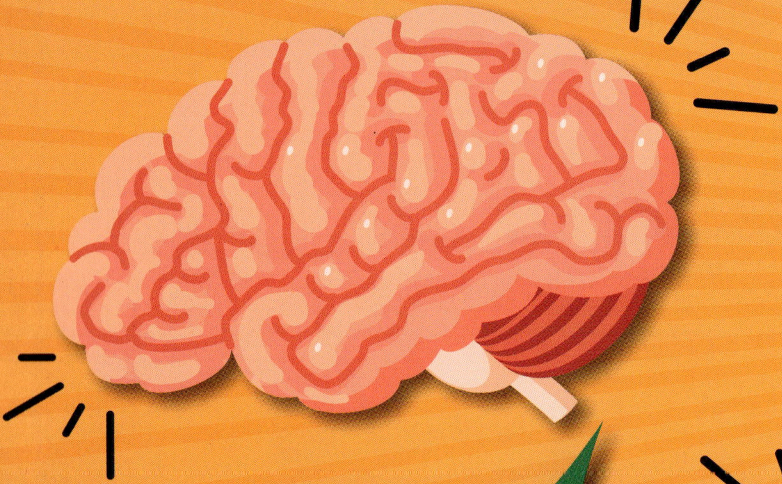

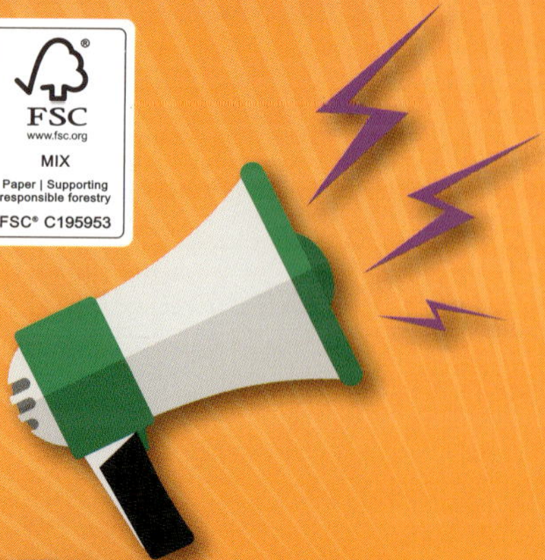

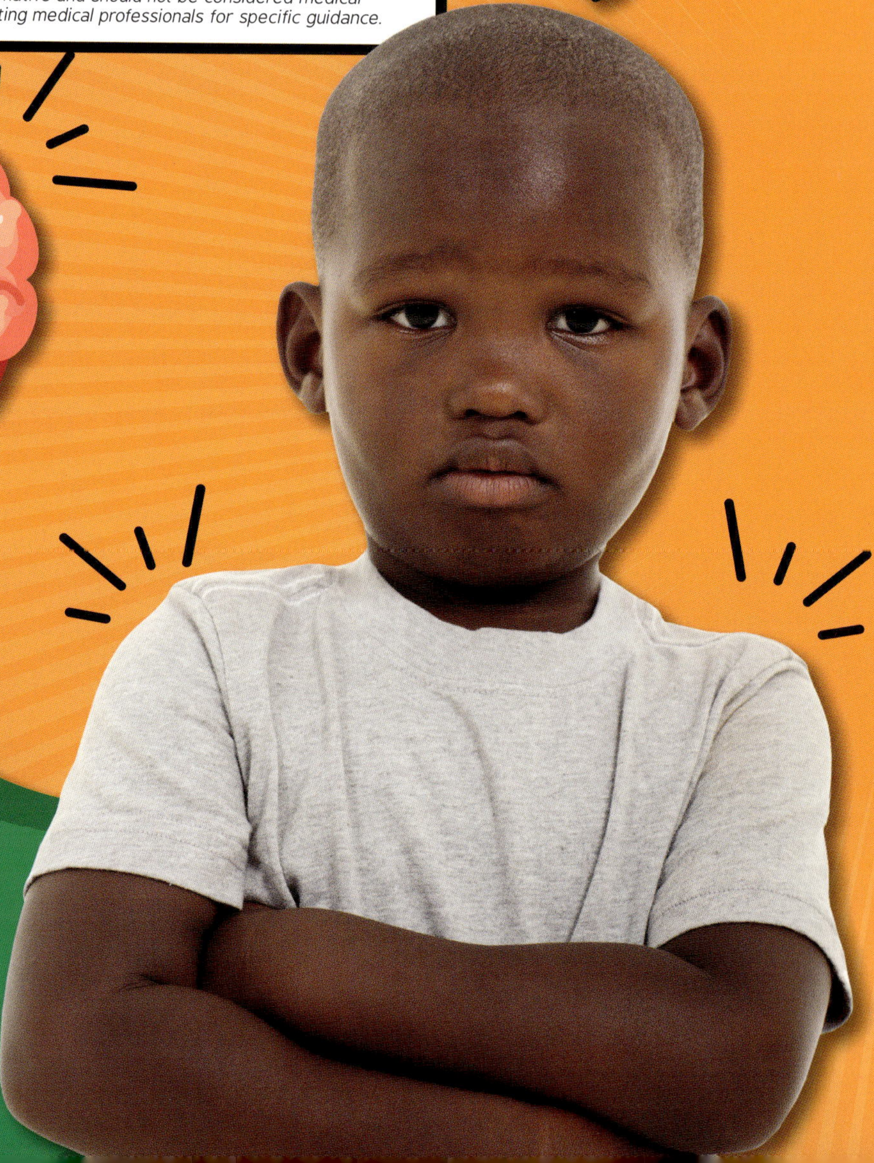

Photo Credits:
Images are courtesy of Shutterstock.com.
With thanks to Getty Images, Thinkstock Photo and iStockphoto.

Front cover – michaeljung, ElephantCastle. 4–5 – Photographee.eu, Prostock-studio, Irina Strelnikova. 6–7 – NOTE OMG, STUDIO GRAND WEB, Syda Productions. 8–9 – Photographee.eu, Yuliya Evstratenko. 10–11 – YanLev, Volurol, ArtFamily. 12–13 – Drazen Zigic, LeManna, Vitali Michkou, Ilike, Nataly Mayak, Anne Richard, Photographee.eu, InesBazdar. 14–15 – pathdoc, Alina Tanya, Stockbusters, wavebreakmedia. 16–17 – Golubovy, Dmitry Lobanov, Zapylaiev Kostiantyn, Ekaterina Pokrovsky, TeodorLazarev, Sergey Novikov, Anatoliy Karlyuk, MIA Studio, Veja, 3445128471. 18–19 – YAKOBCHUK VIACHESLAV, Dubova, kornnphoto. 20–21 – Veja, Tatiana Gordievskaia. 22–23 – Liderina, EZ-Stock Studio.

CONTENTS

PAGE 4	Would You Know What to Do?
PAGE 6	What Is Autism?
PAGE 10	What Is an Autistic Meltdown?
PAGE 12	Triggers
PAGE 14	Rumbling Stage
PAGE 16	Autistic Meltdown
PAGE 18	What Can You Do?
PAGE 20	How We Feel
PAGE 22	What Next?
PAGE 23	Living with Autism
PAGE 24	Glossary and Index

Words that look like this can be found in the glossary on page 24.

WOULD YOU KNOW WHAT TO DO?

Hello! My name is Gary. Have you ever seen an emergency? An emergency is when someone needs help because of something dangerous that is happening. Emergencies sometimes happen when people cannot control what they are doing.

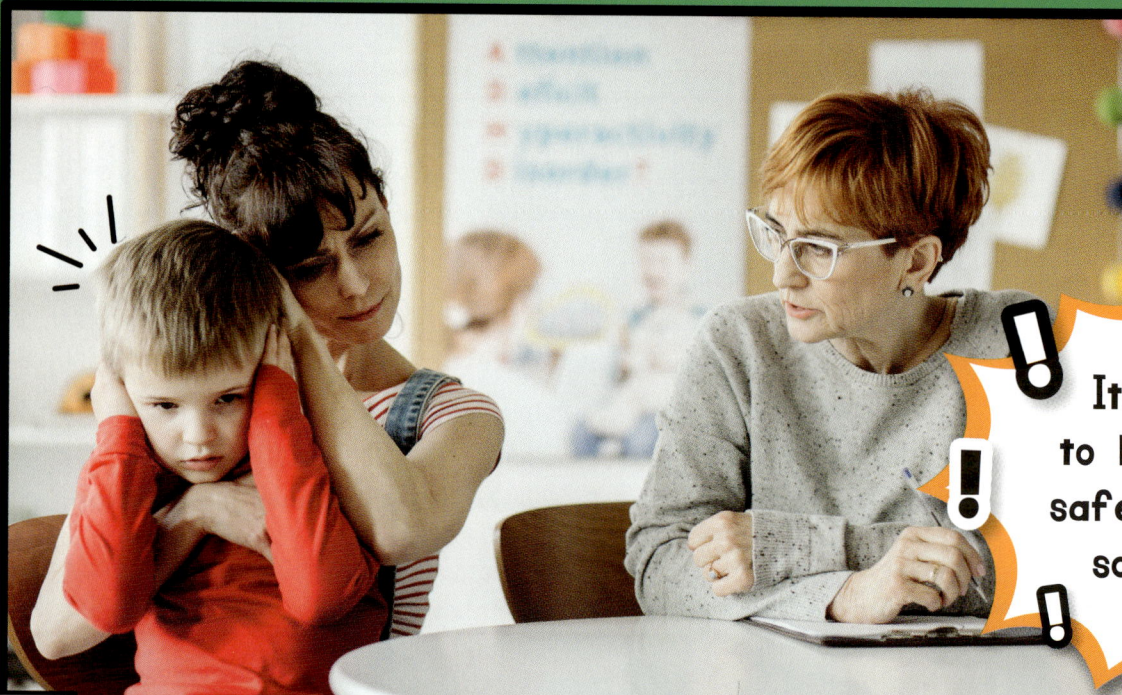

It is important to keep ourselves safe when helping someone else.

People with autism can have an emergency known as an autistic meltdown. They do not need an <u>ambulance</u>, but they do need people who understand meltdowns to help keep them calm and safe.

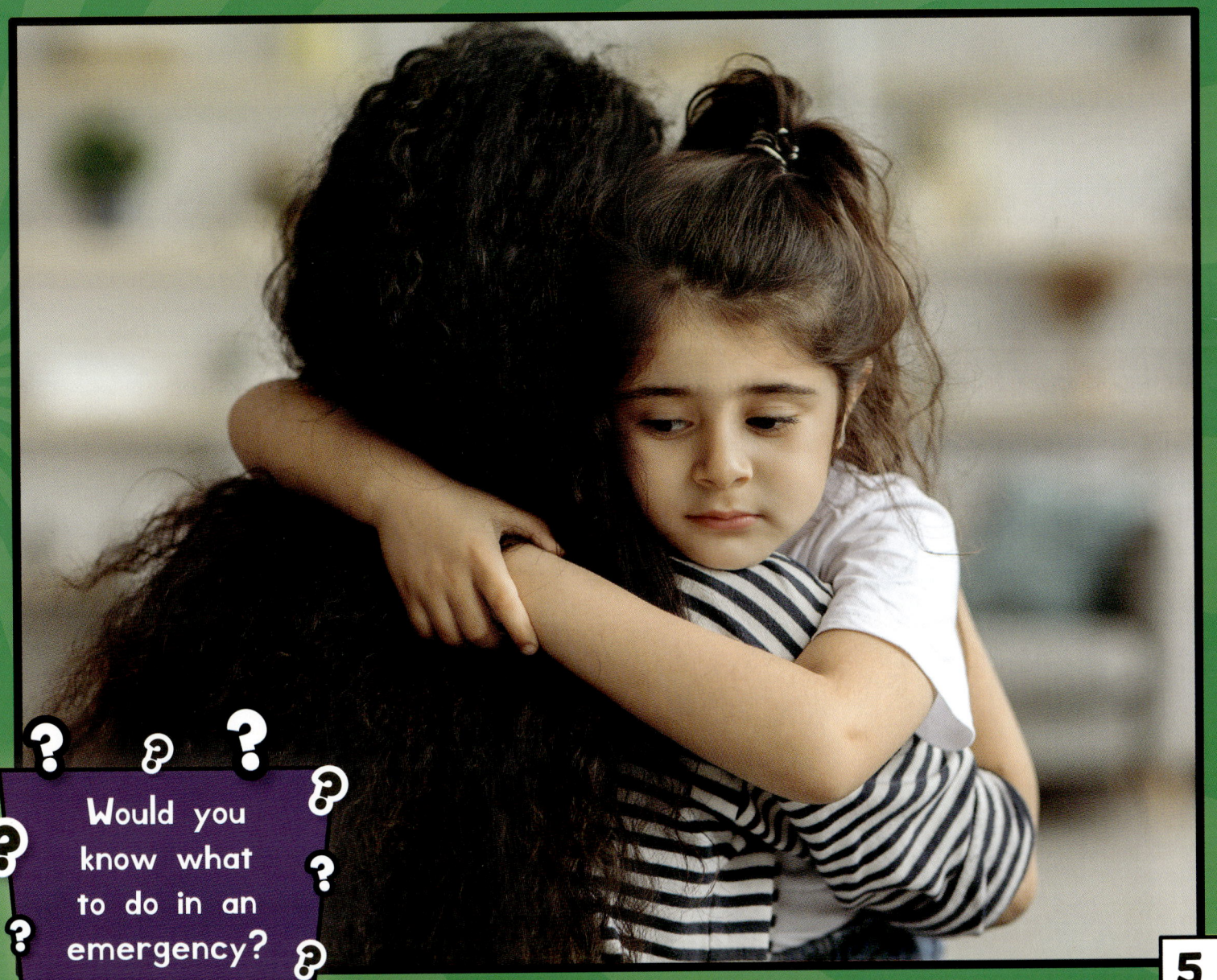

Would you know what to do in an emergency?

WHAT IS AUTISM?

Autism is a difference in someone's brain that changes how they understand the world. People with autism do not have <u>neurotypical</u> brains, which means that they understand things in a different way to most people.

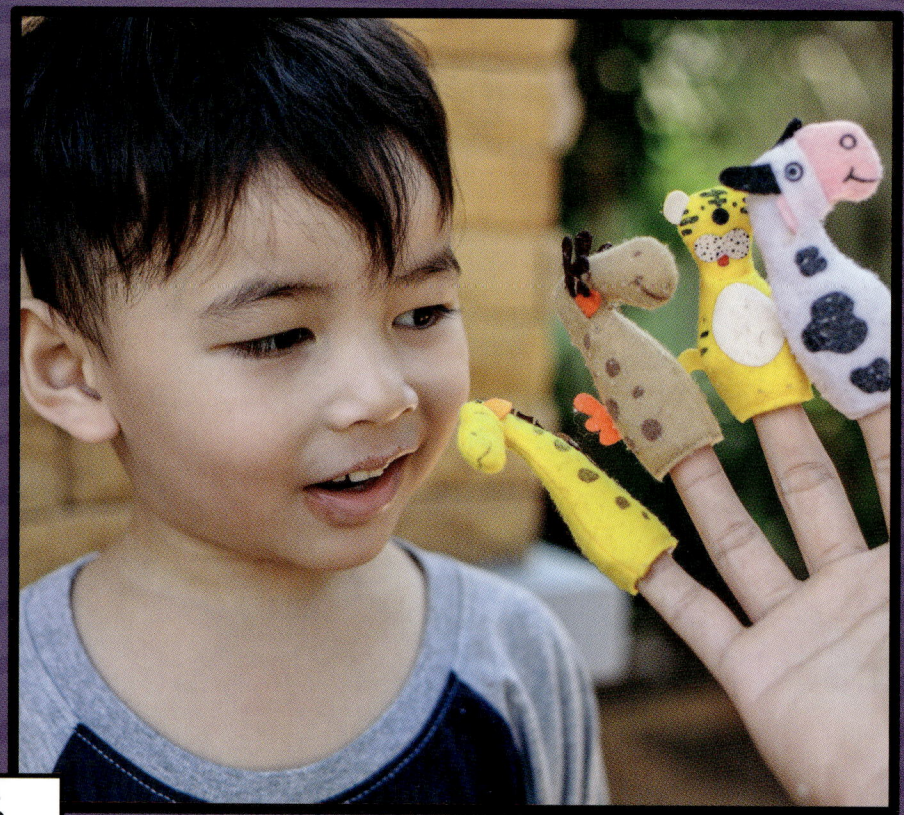
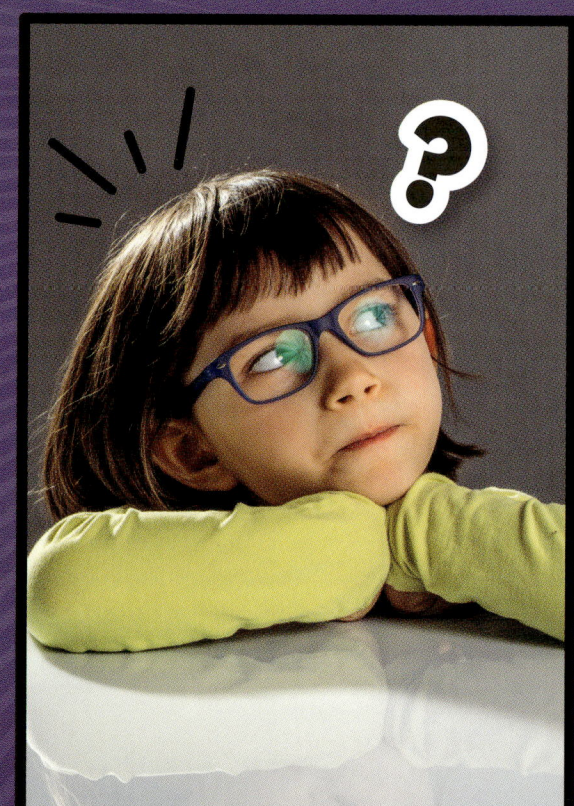

There are many children and adults who have autism. Autism is not the same for everyone. Some people have difficulty being around other people or being in places where there is too much happening.

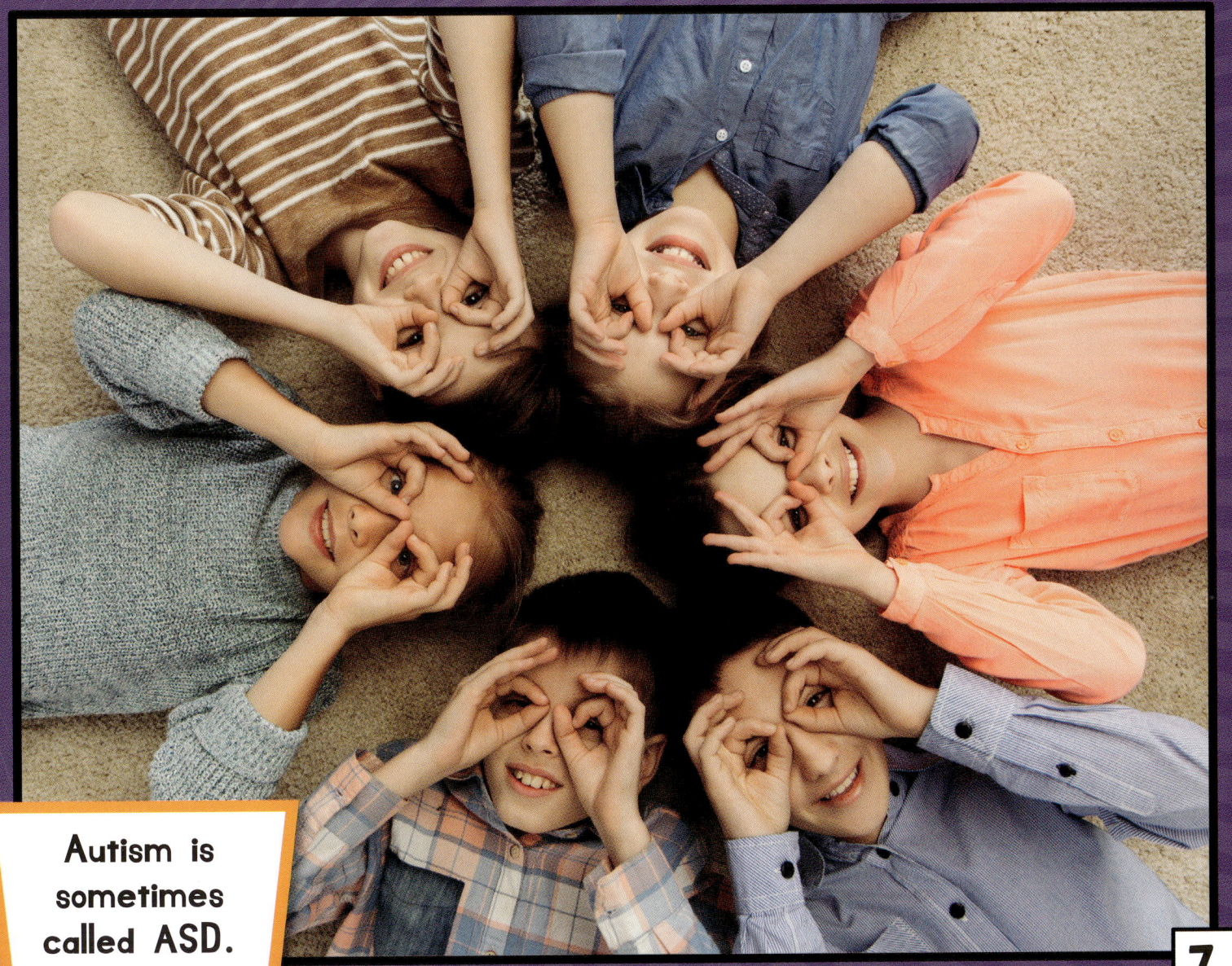

Autism is sometimes called ASD.

It can be hard for some people with autism to <u>communicate</u> in the same way that other people do. Sometimes, they react to things around them more strongly than neurotypical people do.

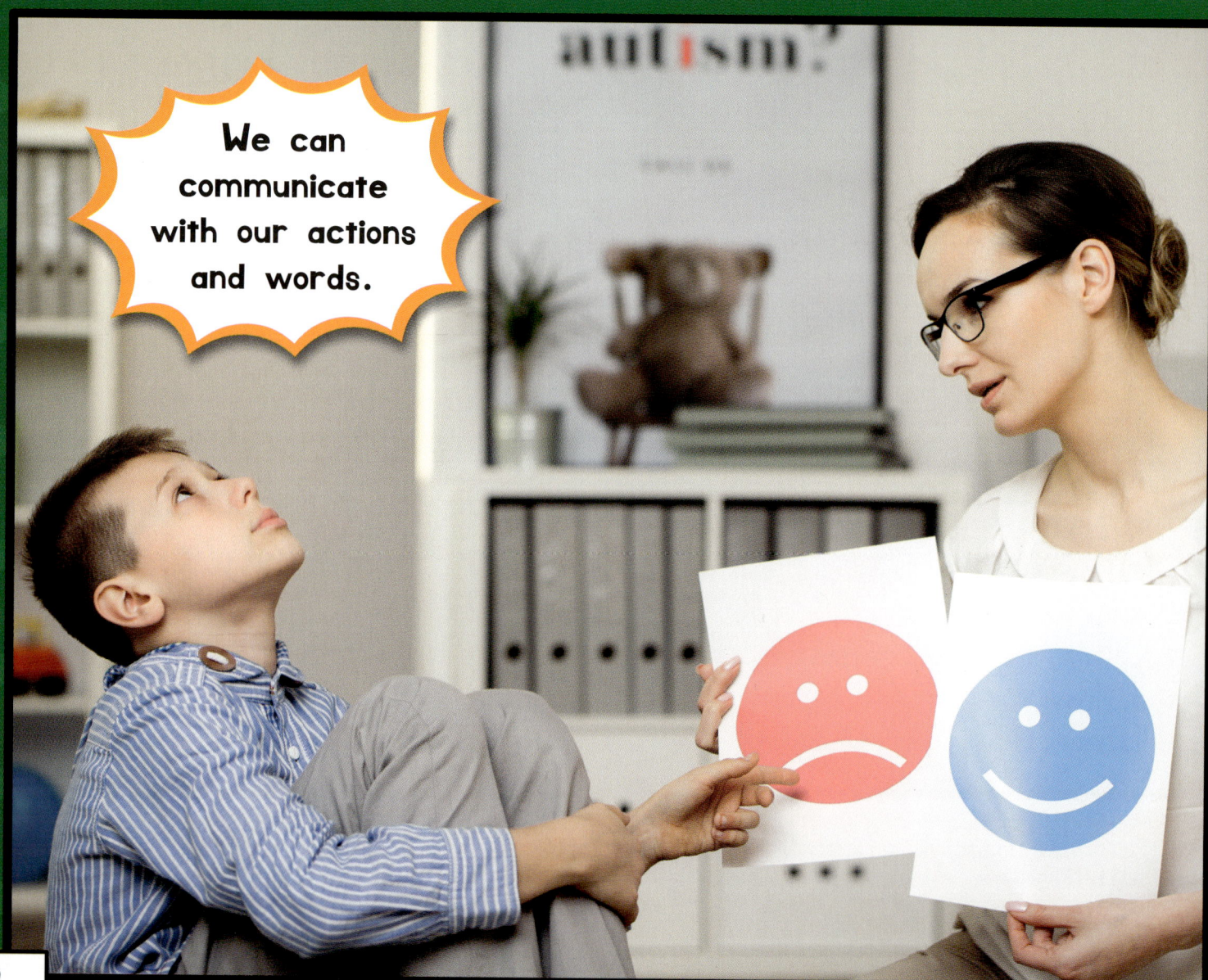

We can communicate with our actions and words.

What is your everyday routine?

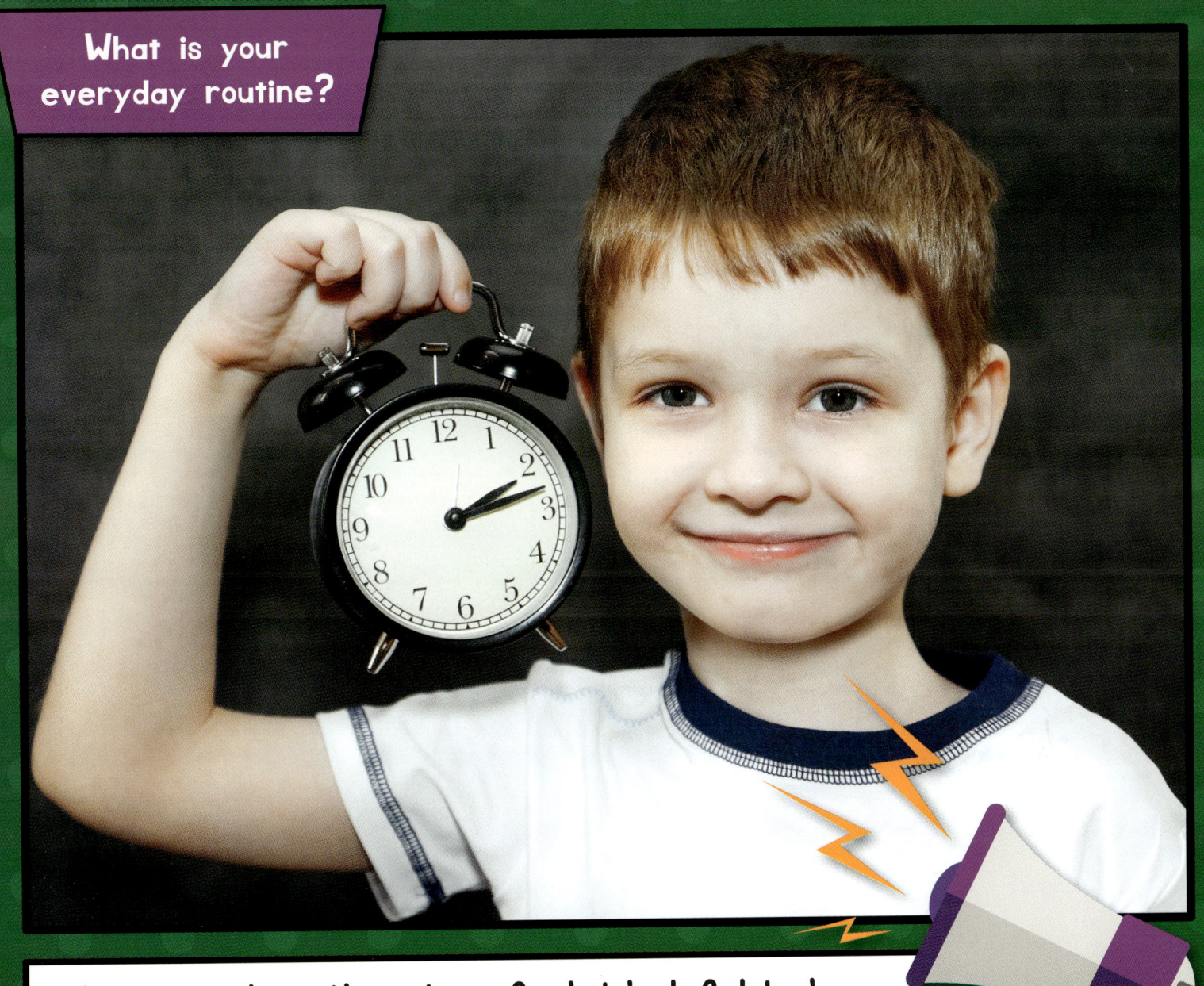

Many people with autism find it helpful to have a routine. A routine is doing things in the same order every day. When things stay the same, it can help someone with autism to feel calm.

WHAT IS AN AUTISTIC MELTDOWN?

People with autism can sometimes react with strong <u>emotions</u> that they cannot control. This is called a meltdown. Meltdowns happen when someone feels <u>anxious</u> and cannot keep calm.

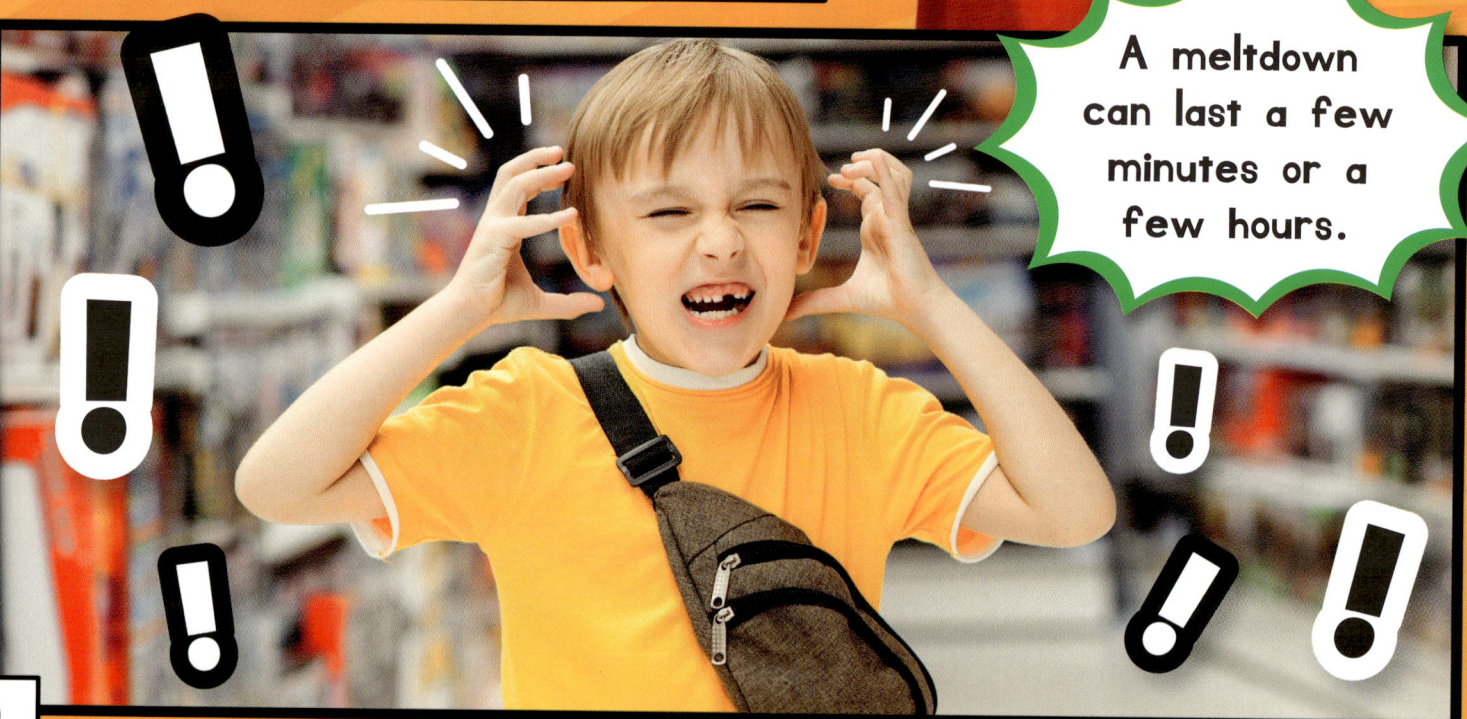

A meltdown can last a few minutes or a few hours.

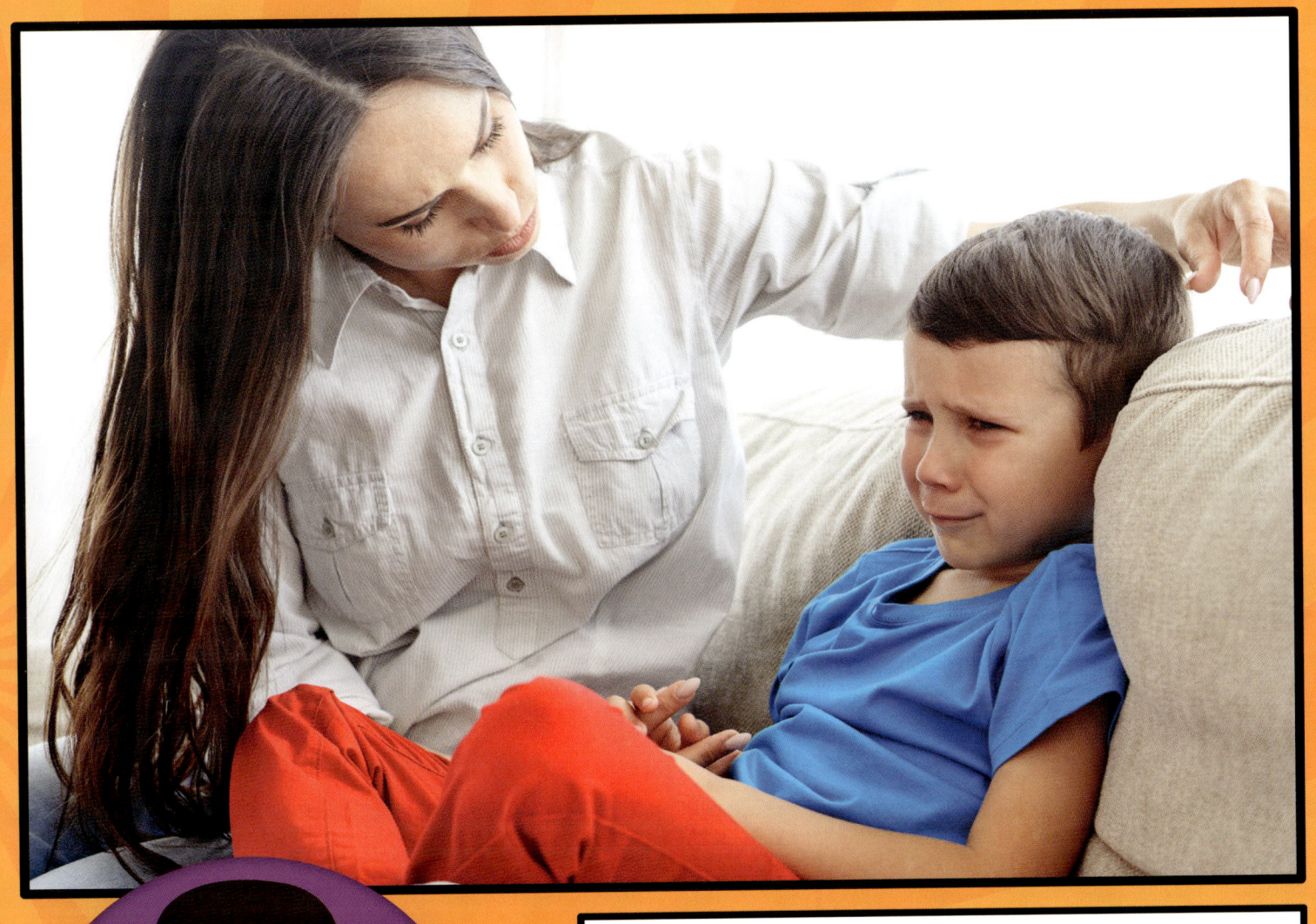

People sometimes think that a meltdown is a <u>temper tantrum</u> or being naughty. Meltdowns are actually a sign that someone with autism is <u>overwhelmed</u> by emotion and needs help calming down.

TRIGGERS

When something causes someone with autism to get very upset, this is called a trigger. Things that seem small to neurotypical people can build up into triggers for people with autism.

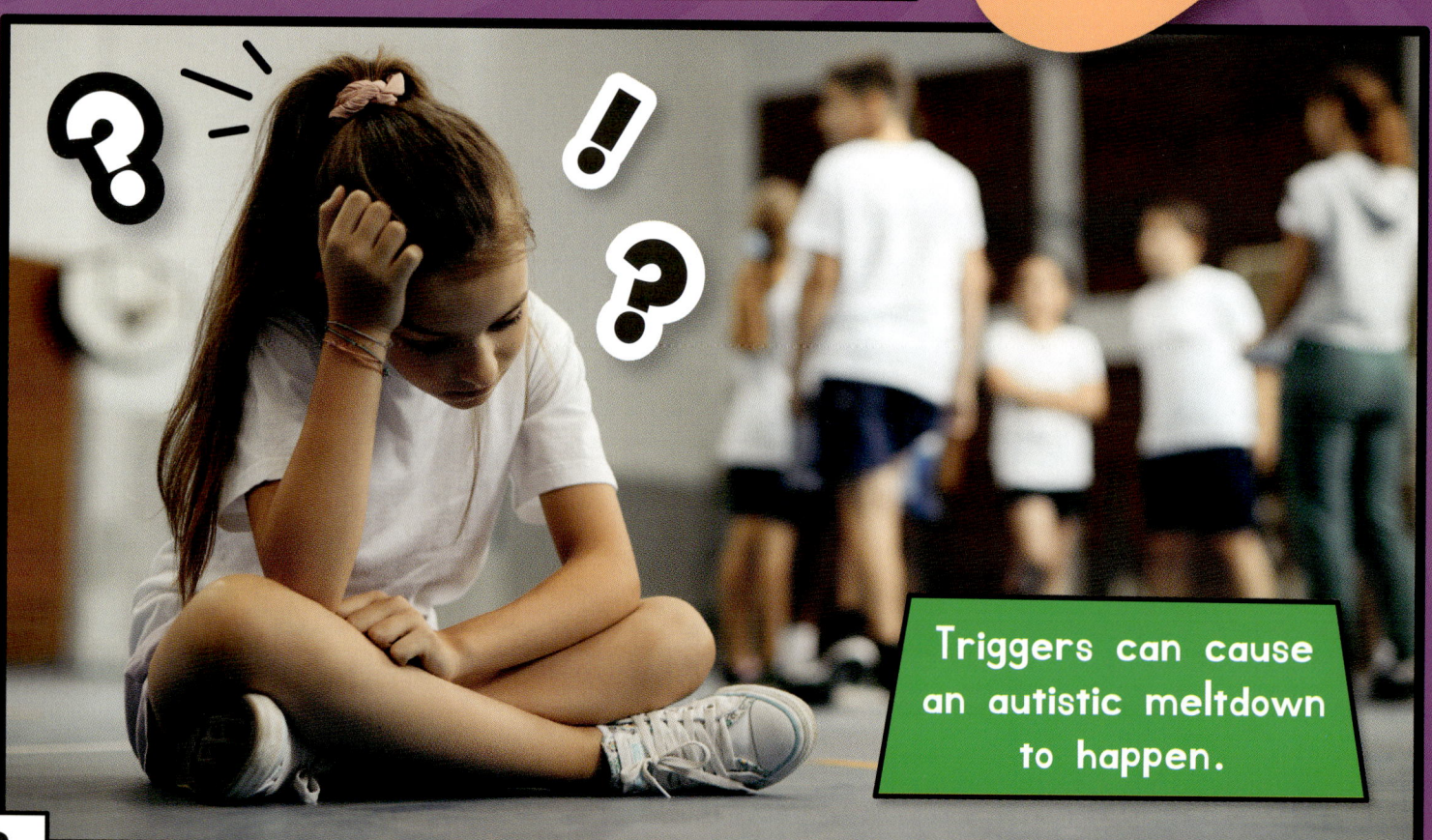

Triggers can cause an autistic meltdown to happen.

Everyone is different, but many people with autism are triggered by...

If you know someone's triggers, you can help them avoid a meltdown.

...STRESSFUL SITUATIONS.

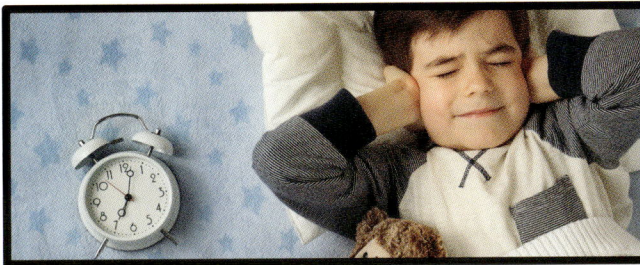
Changes in routine

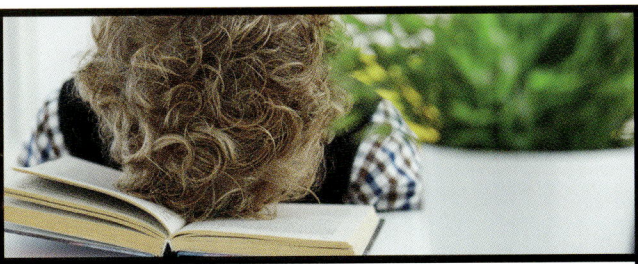
Not understanding something

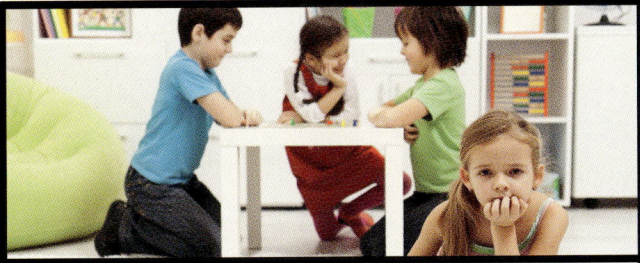
Too many people

...TOO MUCH INFORMATION FROM THE WORLD AROUND THEM.

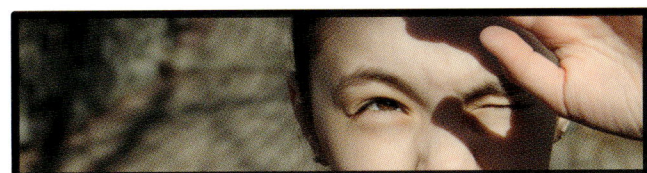
Bright lights

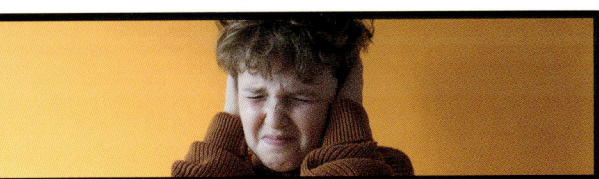
Loud noises

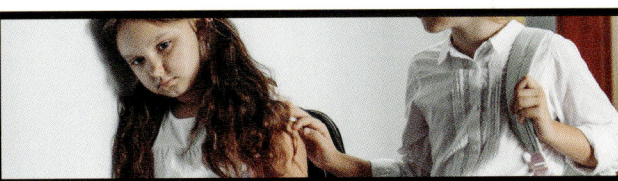
Being touched

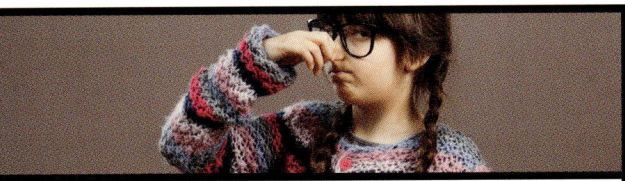
Smells

RUMBLING STAGE

When someone is close to losing control of their emotions, they start to look upset and uncomfortable. This is called the rumbling stage. People with autism might not notice this happening.

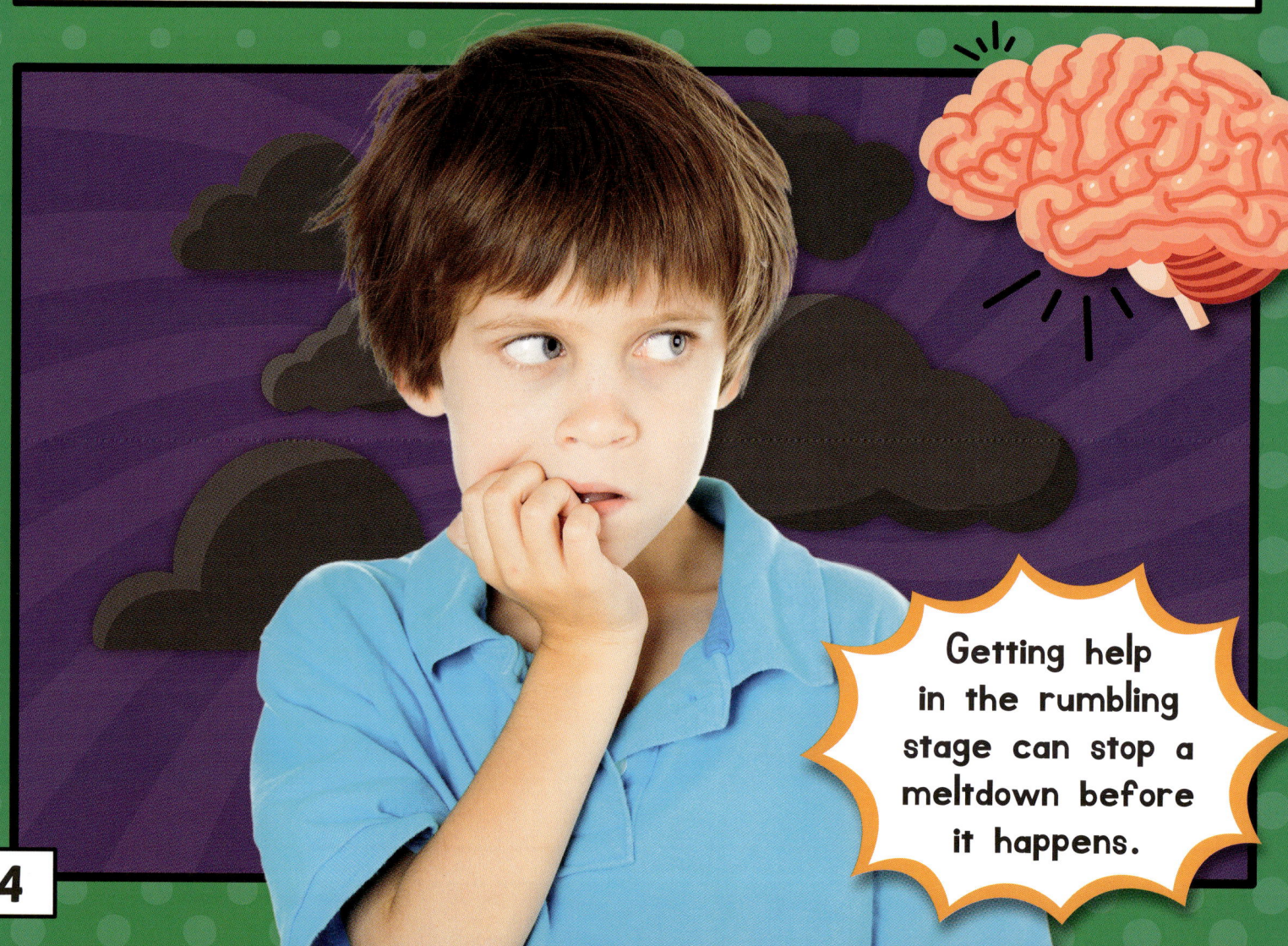

Getting help in the rumbling stage can stop a meltdown before it happens.

In the rumbling stage, someone might look very uncomfortable. They might bite their nails, tap their feet or ask questions over and over. They might try to be alone or move around a lot.

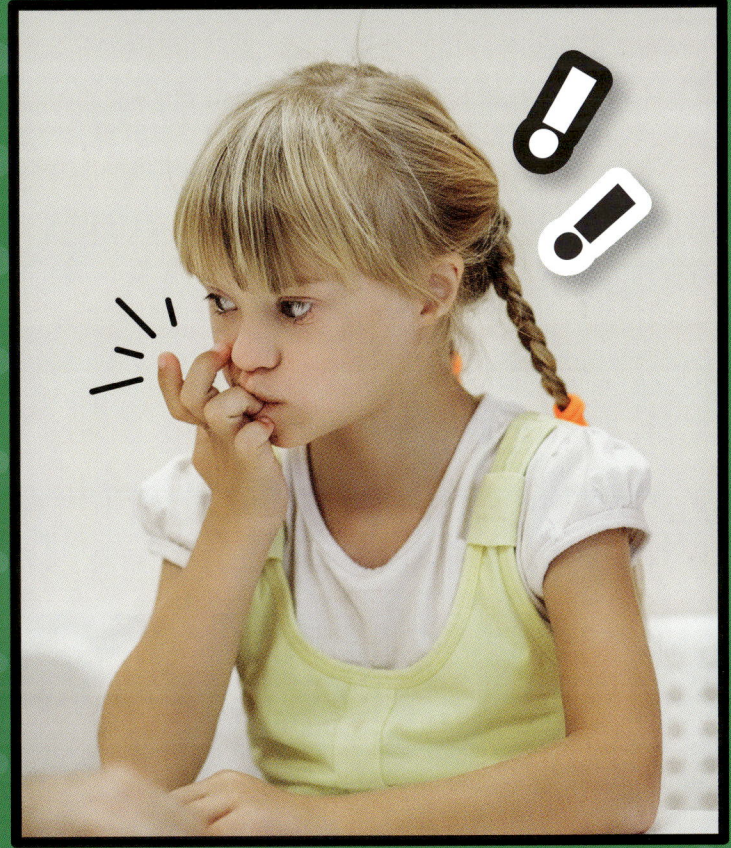

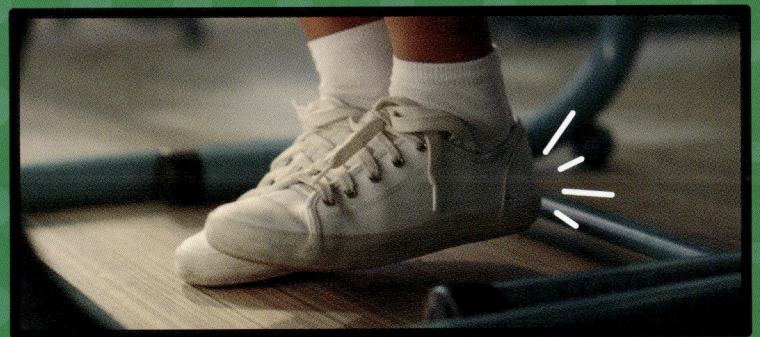

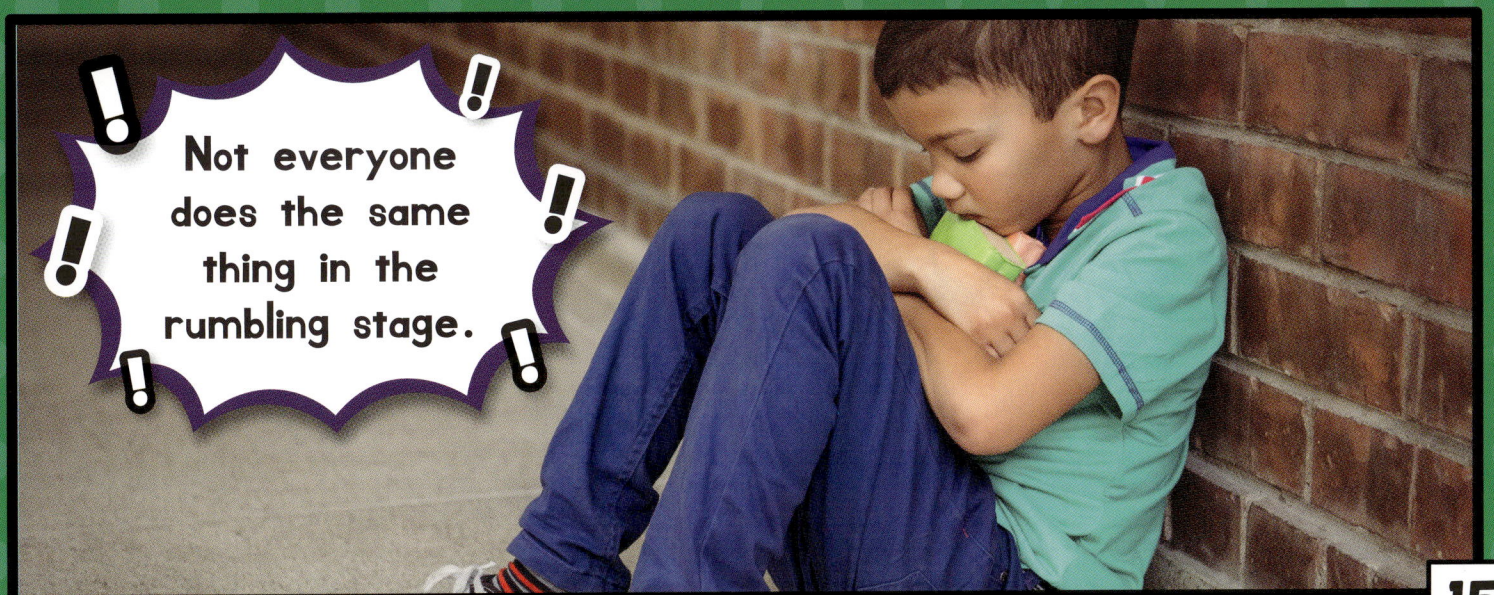

Not everyone does the same thing in the rumbling stage.

AUTISTIC MELTDOWN

If someone with autism does not get help while they are in the rumbling stage, they may have a meltdown. In a meltdown, they are overwhelmed by emotion or information from their <u>senses</u>.

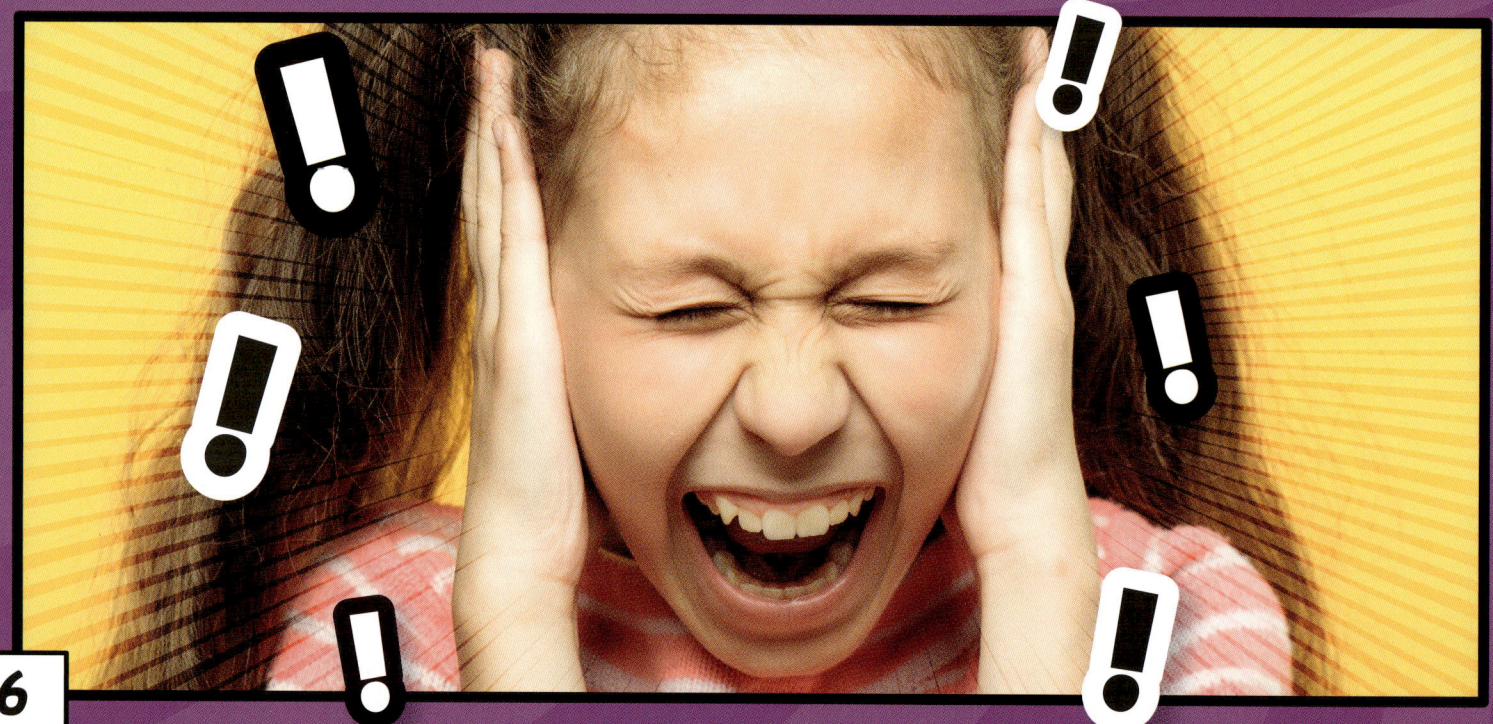

During a meltdown, someone might...

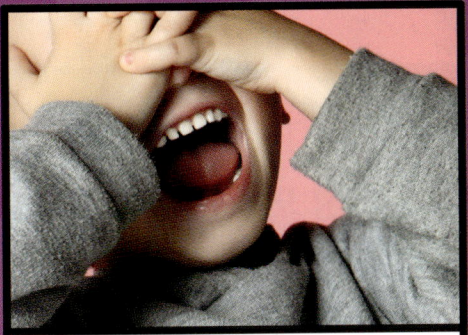
... shout.

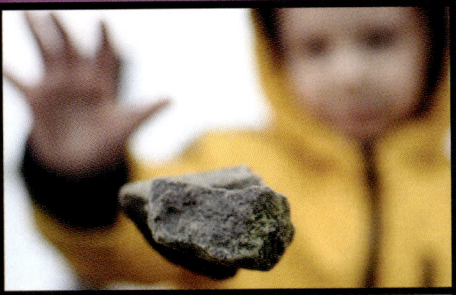
... throw things or flap their arms.

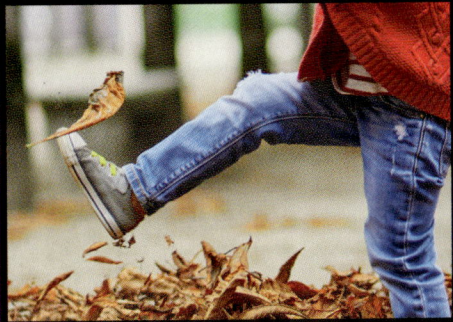
... hit or kick things.

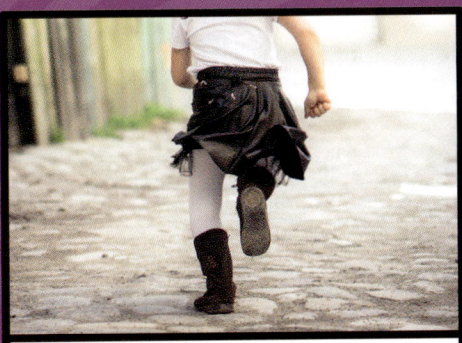
... run.

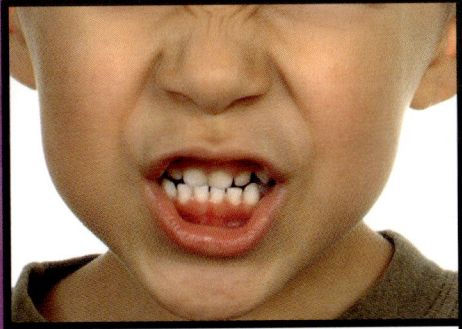
... bite things.

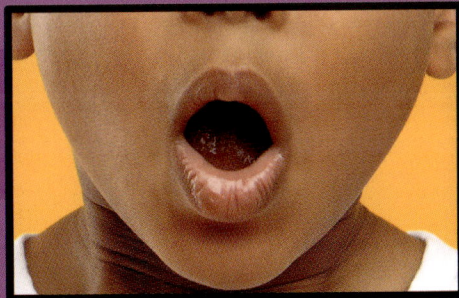
... breathe in and out quickly.

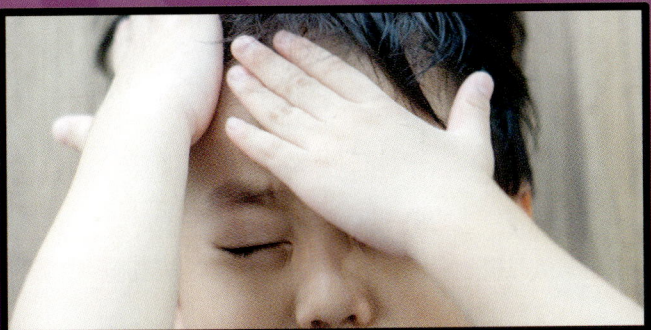
... hit their head.

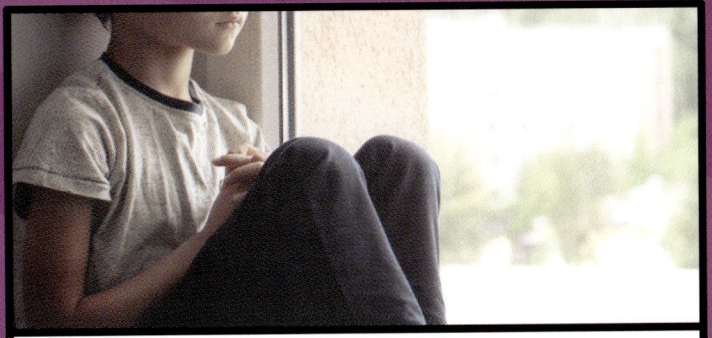
... keep to themselves.

WHAT CAN YOU DO?

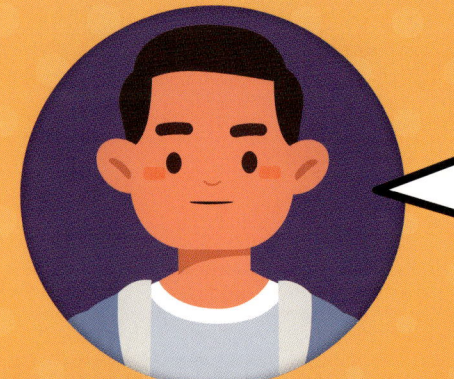

If someone has a meltdown, get a grown-up. Do not try to hug or stop someone who is having a meltdown. It is possible to accidentally hurt them or get hurt yourself when trying to help.

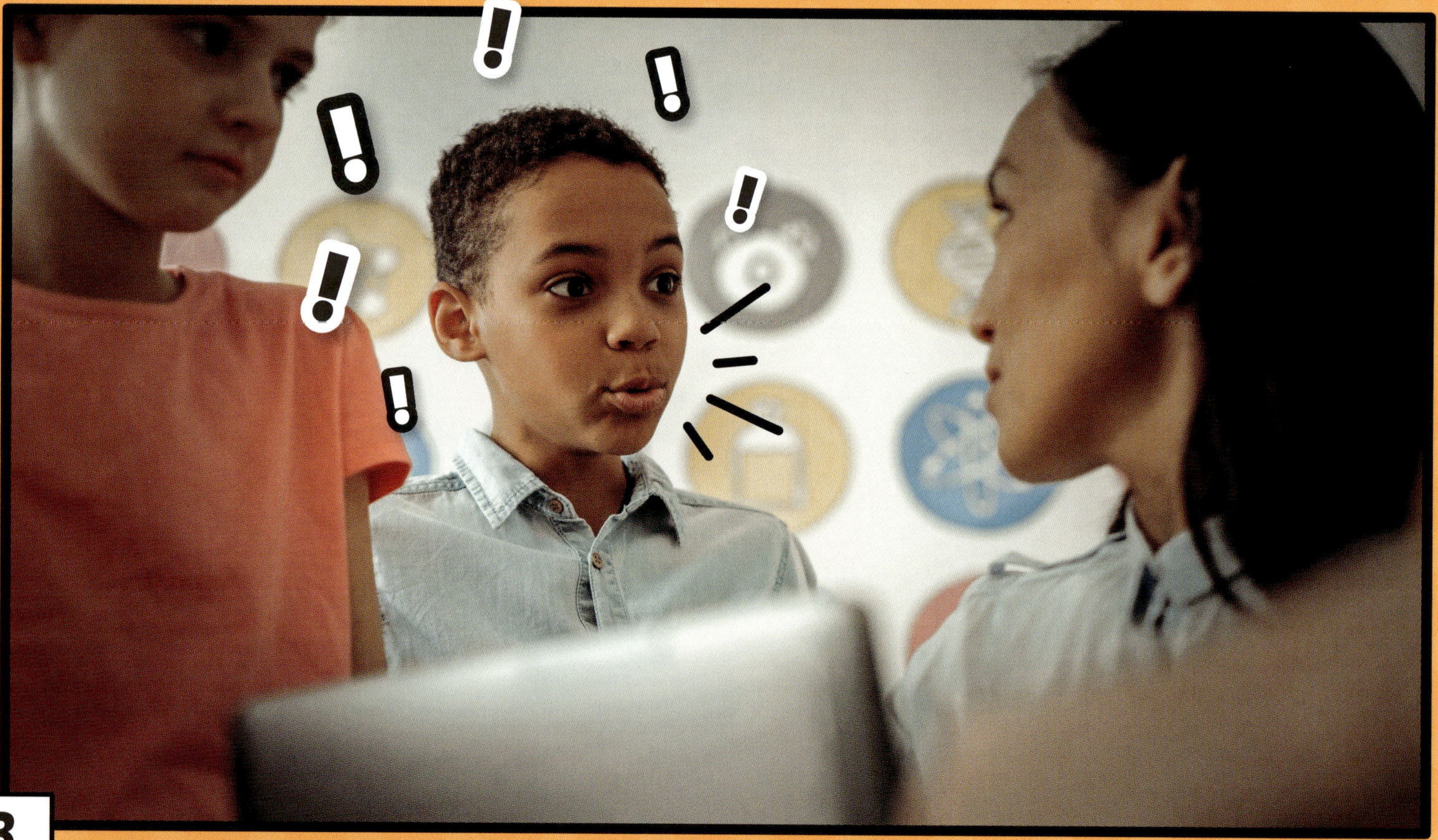

The grown-up might ask you to leave the room or be quieter. This helps to create a safe and calm space for the person with autism. They might turn the lights down or give them headphones to block out sound.

Different people might need different things to calm them.

HOW WE FEEL

A meltdown can be surprising or confusing to see. It is important to stay calm. People who have meltdowns might feel embarrassed and tired when they have calmed down, so be kind.

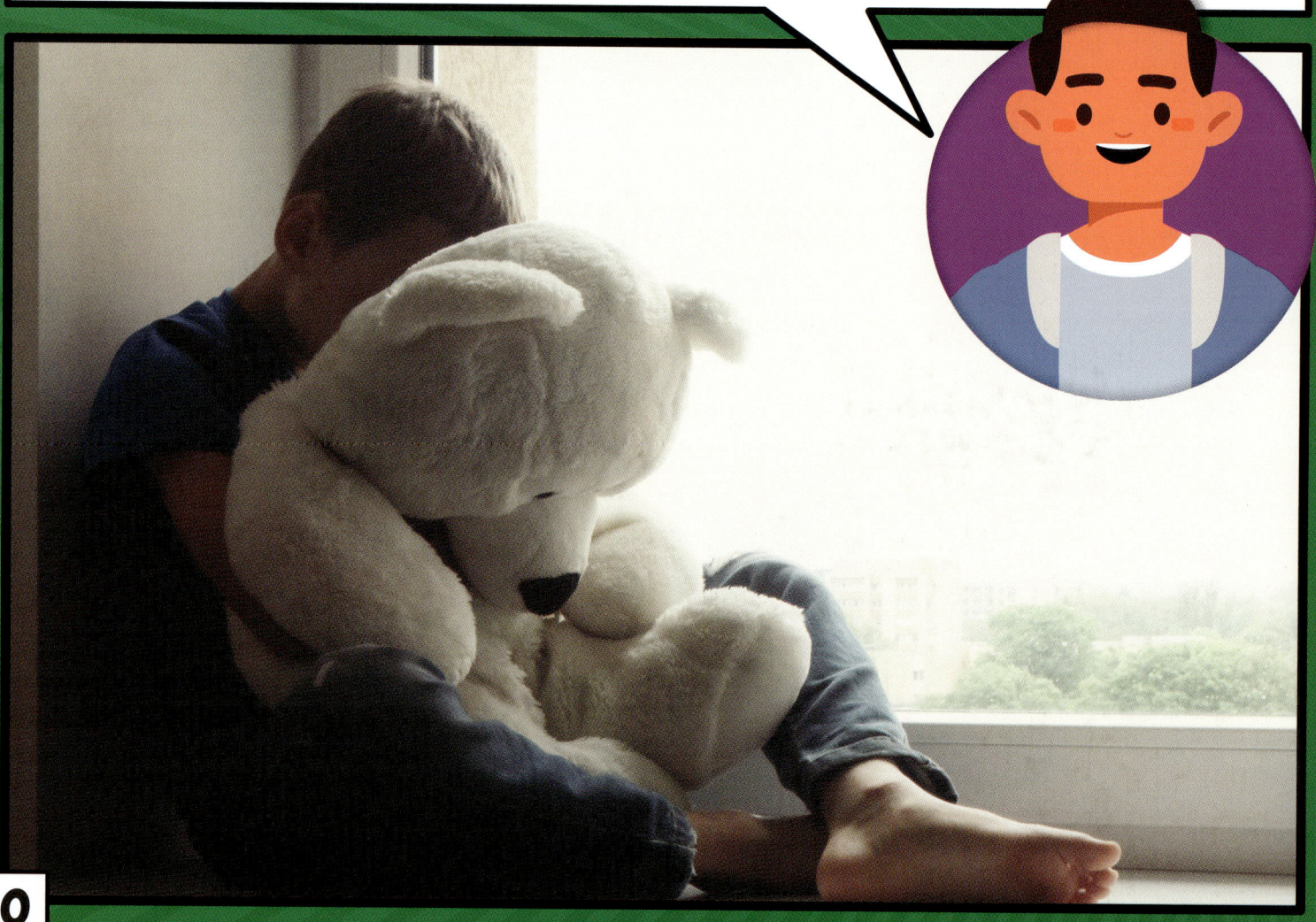

It is never OK to bully someone for being different from us. Everyone is different in their own way, and everyone needs help with different things.

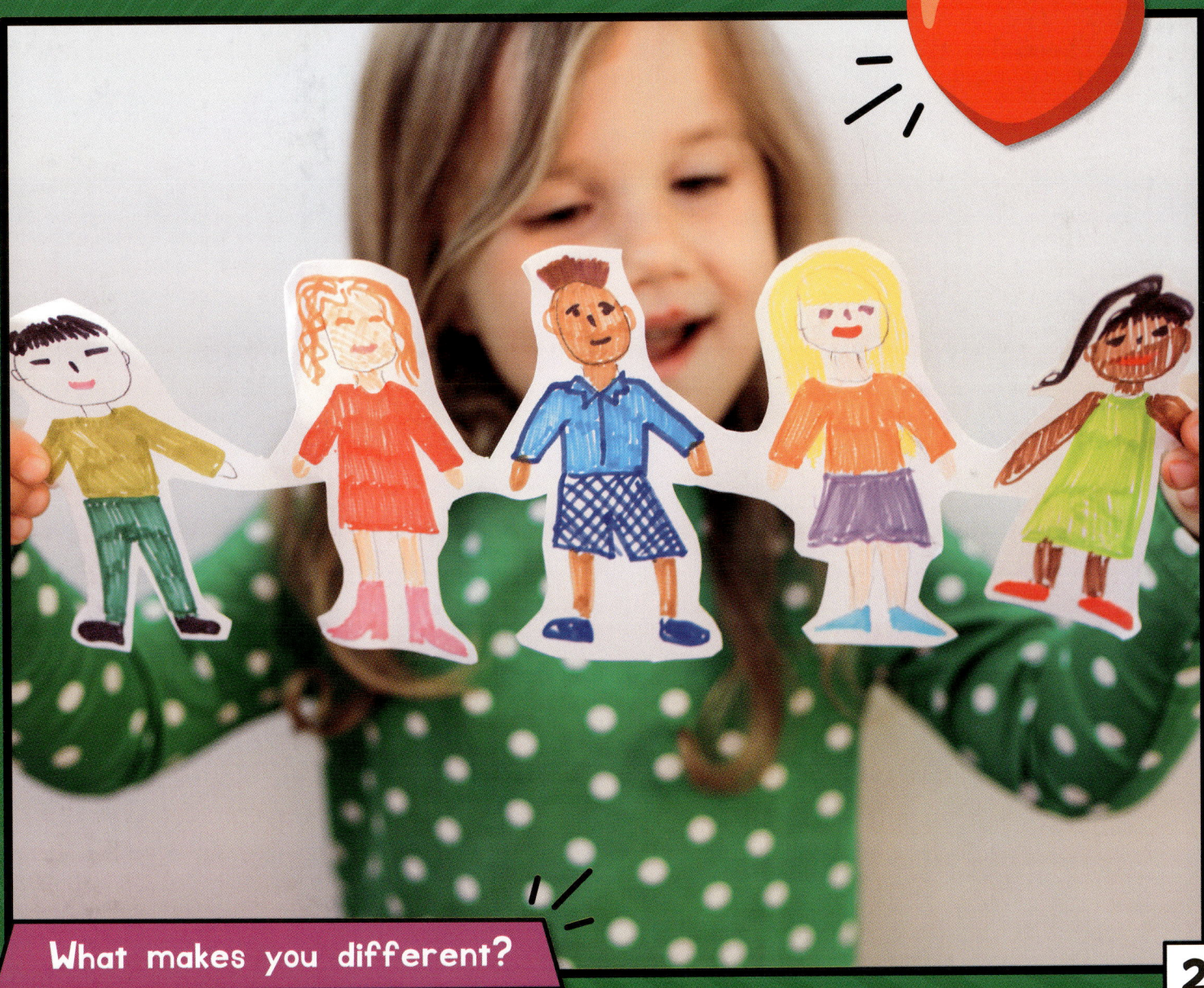

What makes you different?

WHAT NEXT?

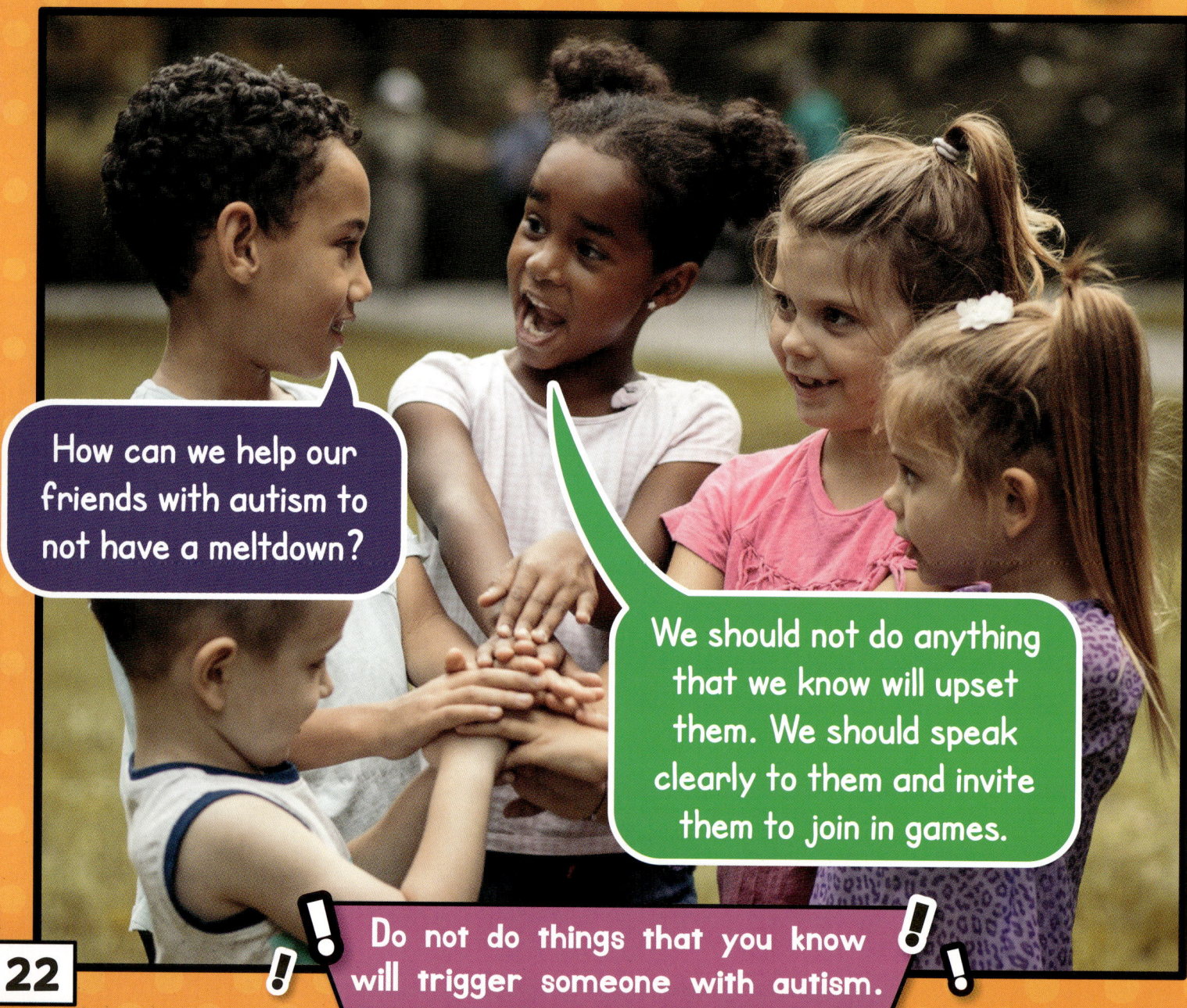

How can we help our friends with autism to not have a meltdown?

We should not do anything that we know will upset them. We should speak clearly to them and invite them to join in games.

Do not do things that you know will trigger someone with autism.

LIVING WITH AUTISM

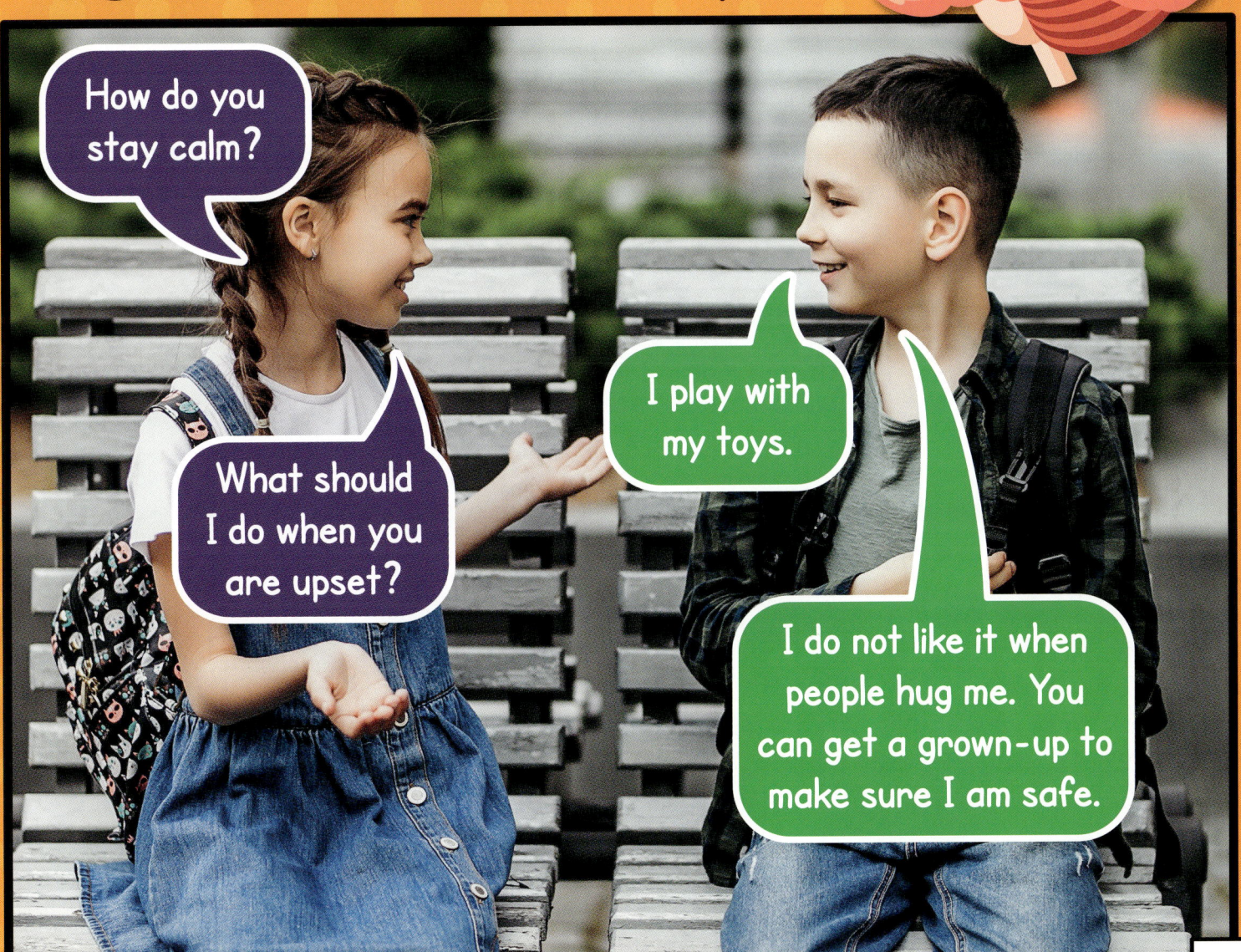

GLOSSARY

AMBULANCE	a vehicle that brings medical help or takes people to a hospital
ANXIOUS	worried
COMMUNICATE	share information with other people
EMOTIONS	feelings such as anger, happiness, fear, or sadness
NEUROTYPICAL	thinking about or experiencing the world in the same way as many other people
OVERWHELMED	feeling too many things at the same time, so that it is hard to know how to deal with everything
SENSES	ways we use our bodies to understand the world, such as by touching, seeing, smelling, hearing and tasting
TEMPER TANTRUM	shouting or doing something naughty because someone is upset

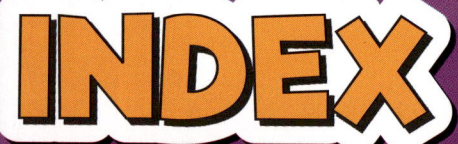

INDEX

BRAINS 6
EMERGENCIES 4–5
GROWN-UPS 18–19, 23
LIGHTS 13, 19
MELTDOWNS 5, 10–14, 16–18, 20, 22
NOISES 13
ROUTINES 9, 13
SENSES 16
SMELLS 13
TOYS 23
TRIGGERS 12–13, 22
WORLD 6, 13